I0756573

AN ISSUE

OF

BLOOD

— JAMIINA —

Copyright © 2019 Jamiina

All rights reserved. No part of this book may be used or reproduced by any means, graphic, electronic, or mechanical, including photocopying, recording, taping or by any information storage retrieval system without the written permission of the author except in the case of brief quotations embodied in critical articles and reviews.

Scripture taken from the King James Version of the Bible

First published in 2019 by WestBow Press

This edition independently published by the author 2020

ISBN: 9798620050871 (paperback)

This book is dedicated to

My Momma, for praying over me at 4 a.m. every morning when she
thought I was asleep
Mose and Toot, family that never gave up on family
My 'Home Girl' LuJuana Brown, for kickin' me in the shins!

~ & ~

Every woman who is 'A CERTAIN WOMAN'

Preface

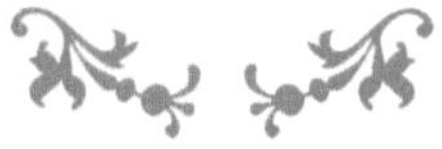

This book is NOT a formal medical report, journal or magazine article, or any other official form of documentation of medicine or medical treatment. This book IS a memoir that records the experience of one woman and of many women everywhere who have faced, and may still be facing, serious health problems and concerns relating to uterine fibroids, abnormal uterine bleeding (AUB) and the female reproductive system.

An Issue of Blood reveals the negative effects these serious health issues have on the families, jobs, social lives and standards of living of these women. It describes the experience and the effects of various medical procedures, such as uterine ablation and hysterectomy, while asking whether these and other serious female reproductive conditions are listed as physical disabilities.

Last, but most important, this book is a testament to the healing virtue, the wise counsel and the specific instructions from the GOD that is Savior and Healer. Moving through HIS people, the Lord brought about complete healing for two women in different times and places. One woman had her experience biblically recorded, and the other has documented her own.

A Certain Woman

'And a certain woman, which had an issue of blood twelve years' (Mark 5:25, King James Version [KJV])

This woman could have been any woman—someone's wife, mother, sister or daughter. She could have been from any socioeconomic background, of any race or color. At the time of the recorded biblical accounts, *Matthew* 9:20–22, *Mark* 5:25–34 and *Luke* 8:43–48, she was someone experiencing a problem that is experienced by many women today. The biblical accounts are short (the account in *Mark* 5:25–34 being the longest) but specific and conclusive. The accounts demonstrate much respect by not recording the personal details of her life. The only description is of her physical condition, how long she had the problem, her efforts to resolve the issue and at last the resolution of it.

The nature of her physical condition was serious enough for it to be described as 'a plague', 'a fountain of blood' and 'a disease'. The meaning of the Hebrew word for 'issue' is 'a gushing fluid' according to *Strong's Exhaustive Concordance*, and this was not the full extent of her problems. We read in the book of *Leviticus* 15:1–30 (KJV) that this woman had to be 'set apart' from her house, family, friends and whatever her daily routine was for seven days—longer if the blood flow persisted beyond seven days.

Please keep in mind, this time of separation was due to a woman of that day having a 'normal period'. Nothing about this poor woman's situation was normal ... nothing.

Twelve years of forced separation from her husband and children (if she had any) had to have been difficult in so many ways. The scriptures state that she 'spent all that she had', or 'all her living', on doctors. She may have been a woman who worked, or maybe the money was coming from her husband. Can you imagine the financial strain, the emotional stress and the humiliation of being treated like an outcast and living with the possible threat of being stoned and going from one doctor to the next and being told, 'I can't help you'? This woman probably had to travel inconspicuously because she was supposed to be separated from everybody. Being called 'a certain woman' in the Bible leads me to think that her name was omitted to protect her and her family from embarrassment and the hundreds of millions of eyes that would read those scriptures. I wonder how she could avoid being barred from the public place where everyone was gathering around Jesus and move through the crowd to get to HIM. I believe Luke, as a physician, was the only person outside of her family who knew she was plagued by this condition. I also believe Luke may have been one of the doctors who examined her. For this 'certain woman', every year the condition got worse. She must have been weak, bowed over and in pain ALL the time.

My Experience

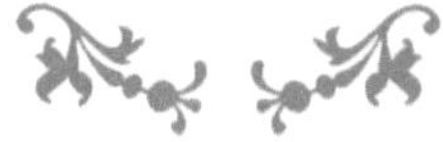

At the time of **THIS** writing, 'a certain woman' was I in the twentieth and twenty-first centuries. And like the 'certain woman' of the biblical account, Jesus was my solution as well. While many of you may think this is coincidental, I say it is nothing short of AMAZING and that it more than confirms *Hebrews* 13:8: *'Jesus Christ the same yesterday, and to day, and for ever'* (KJV). Twelve years is a long time to suffer from any kind of infirmity, affliction or disease, and the loss of blood is critical. My time of suffering this debilitating infirmity was the same. I did not separate myself as required or practiced in the Mosaic laws of the Bible. By the very nature of the problem, the pain, the irritability and the abnormal and constant bleeding, I was automatically separated from outdoor events, my husband and to a small degree my children.

I was anemic from the age of eleven, which is also exactly the time puberty sprung like spring—but there was nothing flowery about it. Puberty sprung a bloody leak. My first menstrual cycle was horrible. I thought I was dying. I was into my eleventh year by six months. It was late spring, and like any eleven-year-old I had been outside with the rest of the kids on the block, having the time of my life looking crisp, clean and happy. The cramping pain came suddenly. I thought I had eaten a rotten apple or some bad candy. The pain increased to the point I became dizzy. I went to my bedroom where I just rolled around, leaning on the side of the bed. I was in too much pain to get in the bed. By this time my Mom had come in and I managed to tell her between groans and the room spinning around that my stomach was hurting. She gave me a hot cup of tea and a children's aspirin and put me to bed with a hot water bottle on my stomach. Twenty minutes after she left me with some comfort, I rushed to the bathroom with blood trailing everywhere. That is how it happened to me. I was glad it happened at home.

That is when I started taking liquid ferrous sulfate, the chemical name for an iron compound used to treat anemic or low blood, along with my vitamins. I was the only one of my siblings taking iron. From the age of eleven onward, I was always tired and the older I got the more tired I became.

All of the extracurricular activities I participated in were short lived because of this. I no longer felt crisp, clean or happy, and to make matters worse feminine hygiene products were not designed as they are now. All feminine hygiene products bore the cumbersome design of male ingenuity, None of them were convenient especially from a child's perspective. From the beginning my cycles were heavy. When my cycles ended I would 'return to normal'. Outside of a regular wellness physical and childhood vaccinations for measles, mumps, chicken pox and rubella, no doctors were involved ... yet.

Every female is different. Because I felt like I was the only girl my age going through this (yes, I thought that), I wondered about my female grade school peers. Nobody ever talked about having your cycle. I wondered if any of them were also feeling self-conscious, isolated and embarrassed. It was not until I was ending sixth grade that I found out I was not the only girl in class having this problem. Other girls were having 'accidents'. 'Accidents' happened when you got your first menstrual cycle. You never knew when or where this would happen. With no way to change your clothes, you simply tied a jacket around you (if you had one). The teacher took you to the nurse for a crash course in how to wear a maxi pad. After you cleaned up and washed your clothes (there were washers and dryers for home economics classes), your parents picked you up and nobody saw you at school for at least two days. I was embarrassed and felt bad for my female classmates and myself.

I was angry too, because I had a lot of questions I did not know how or whom to ask. Remember, at that time (the early 1970s) having your period was NOT discussed in grade school, even though we were taking physical education (PE) and health classes.

I was already a shy and quiet person. I wanted to be on my best behavior especially in school. Having a period turned a naturally timid girl into a very self-conscious woman. As long as I experienced having a cycle, I would always be fearful of 'accidents'. There were ALWAYS 'accidents' even as an adult and more often as an adult, in public or private settings. I was always checking my clothes if my body temperature changed.

Time and Change

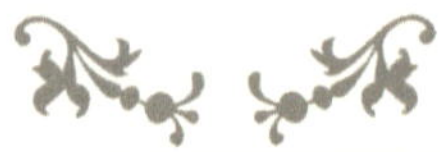

Turning thirty was indeed 'turning'. I knew immediately my body was changing, although there were no delayed internal indicators showing any outward signs of my body changing. Change just happened. Natural change, of course—but then something different. It felt the same way a car feels when you have four-wheel drive and you downshift: you feel the transmission react to the shifting but the car continues to operate smoothly if the transmission is good. When this physical change took place my mind changed with it. Having heard other women talking about how their bodies changed when they reached their thirties, I did not give this information much consideration. When I experienced all this *changing,* my mind and my thought processes were very different in terms of how I handled day-to-day activities. I remember before thirty I would lift something heavy without thinking about it. Nothing that required the strength of a man, mind you. I would effortlessly grab a box full of books (you know this is heavy) and just toss it wherever I wanted it to be. I remember stacking corners of boxes and re-arranging them at any time, all at the snap of my fingers.

My mother tried telling me that females, young or older, were not physically built to lift heavy objects consistently. I would laugh and say, 'Well Mamma, what are women supposed to do when we either don't have a man or can't find one?' Of course my Momma ALWAYS had the last word: 'You drag it or leave it where it is.' I would laugh and wait until she left the room, snap my fingers—and voila, the box was moved!

(Maybe I should have tried blinking like a genie.) Turning thirty confirmed what Mamma had said. Ha!

Turning thirty stopped me from 'snapping' boxes and stacking corners. I shifted to dragging them or putting them on rolling carts and moving them all at once or not at all.

By this time, I was married ... with children. I was so busy taking care of my family and other things that I forgot to take care of me. Now ladies, we all know that it is an unfortunate but common occurrence for many of us to neglect our self-care. Not taking care of myself, not getting regular checkups helped propel the affliction of irregular periods to the horror of AUB.

During my thirties my cramping became so bad I would become extremely nauseated, light-headed and dizzy. Sweat would drip from my hair and require the use of a towel. When I slept my pillows would be soaked. I stopped buying cloth pillows and slept with huge bath towels under my head.

Work and the Public

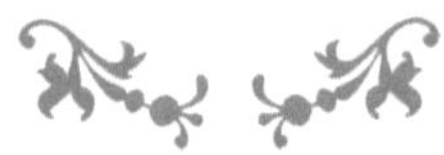

The Lord blessed me to be able to stay home until my children started school. Moving from my home environment to a full-time or overtime work environment was physically shocking to my body. I started working two jobs, and both jobs were in manufacturing and warehouse positions for global manufacturing companies. At this point, I was able to throw boxes for a paycheck after my children started attending school. Having great benefits and getting regular physicals became top priorities. I counted my blessings with gratitude and worked harder to prove to GOD and man (my employers) my worthiness.

The work that I did was not physically demanding. I did not do any heavy lifting, but I did lift small items—bending, stooping, climbing stairs and ladders. Constantly walking the length of the large warehouse areas put my physical condition on level two of getting worse. Increased physical movement was much more demanding than bending to pick up toys scattered around my children's bedrooms.

At home, there was air-conditioning. In these warehouses you had air-conditioning only in certain departments and if you were not assigned to work in these air-conditioned areas you were just miserable. I do have to admit that these employers had huge industrial fans that blew cool air so it was not as bad as some warehouse positions. However, I should have been refrigerated.

The jolting pain I was experiencing before I went to work outside my home happened with increased frequency. This pain would stop me from doing anything until it eased. I knew I was on the second level of a worsening situation the day I was assigned to an air-conditioned area. This assignment came during a holiday and peak summer season. The area was a sterile area, which meant I had to wear a long-sleeved lab jacket or smock with gloves and a hair net. ***Extra clothes*** ... so much for air-conditioning.

This day started with me already tired because of managing two jobs and the family (I was doing *the most*), and my cycle was approaching. I came to work wishing I were still at home. My skin got tight all over and I started complaining about everything. Things I normally paid no attention to were now the focus of my attention. I felt myself frowning. Everyone who knew me was used to me being a very optimistic person most of the time. (I am still the same person.) One of my co-workers said my facial expression resembled a black cloud. I *felt* like a black cloud filled with a storm of radical hormones on their irregular threshold of spilling over to my embarrassment. At level two things were normal enough that my body would send my brain these warnings before the 'fall-out' of any public embarrassment. Looking back, I should have been grateful. I remember leaning against a wall telling somebody, I wish I could walk in the front door and out the back and still get paid. They laughed. I was so serious.

The sterile department of this warehouse was known as line one. Line one, an air-conditioned area was the size of two football fields. There were automatic conveyors moving at varying speeds, depending on product demand. Nobody came to this department unless they were assigned because there was product demand. There was product demand at peak season. No products were on the conveyors and everybody was posted up in the hallway waiting.

Because I was new to Line one, I got a quick run down of how the line worked and what my position was on the line. Everybody rotated through various assigned duties. The products started coming down the conveyors. It was 9 a.m. when I got to my first position and the conveyor continued at a moderate pace. The jolting pain started. By 2 p.m. rotation had taken place six times and I was so miserable. My breathing got short as the jolting increased but because I was on this line, I could not get up and take an extra break. The speed of the line increased. I was now in the flow of my duties and I knew what to do on each rotation.

During the last hours of work, on the last rotation I took my place at the conveyor and the entire room felt as though it was spinning. Sweat broke out all over me. My clothes were wet through and so were the palms of my hands inside those tormenting gloves.

Nausea struck me. I leaned over almost uncontrollably toward the moving lines. I wanted to hurl but did not. I regrouped and sat up straight. This episode backed the work and product up and we all had to stay an extra thirty minutes. Nobody said anything, everybody kept working. Another series of jolts and this time I stood up. Everything came as before—the sweat, the nausea, the blinding headache—but this time after standing up (I had been sitting on a very high stool) I became dizzy. Blood gushed *and* I threw up in this STERILE area.

The last thing I remembered was crawling on the floor trying to get through those horrible plastic strips that covered the doorway and get out of the product area. Hands, voices, the company nurse and my husband were visible blurs. I was wrapped in something soft and white that smelled like hospital antiseptic and was sleepy beyond truth. My husband later told me all the department lines were shut down ... in PEAK SEASON. This was the unfortunate start of every other public embarrassment relating to this condition for the next several years.

As you can probably imagine, I did not go back to either warehouse job. I was on my husband's insurance, so thankfully I was covered medically. I resigned by proxy. My husband was the proxy. Afterwards I worked a series of part-time seasonal positions during the fall and winter holiday seasons. My husband and children were comfortable with this for the obvious reasons. The short work schedule assured me (or so I thought) that everything would go well and without *incident*—and it did. There were no embarrassing moments, ever, during those small seasonal jobs. I was still at level two. My iron dosage was increased and I started taking maximum-strength migraine medicine to diminish the jolts of pain down to 'jilts'. But I enjoyed having my own income and decided I was ready to return to work full time.

Through the Working Class

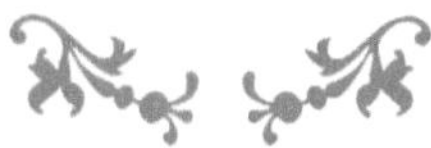

This time I prayed for a job that did not involve manual labor and the Lord blessed me with my first corporate office job. This was in the field of Information Technology. This business was a conglomerate. At the time, the ratio of men to women in the IT job market was unbalanced. That was my first experience with my new IT job.

Being assigned to the micro-systems department as a help-desk specialist was easy enough. I wasn't lifting anything, I wasn't working two jobs and I didn't have to work overtime. I was in employment heaven. I thanked the Lord.

I was introduced to the department as the second of two women, working with seven men. I won't go into the details of the working environment at this job because that is another book. Everything that was bad about my physical condition was 'quarantined' or should I say, without cruel and shameful incident—until we started to approach Y2K. The rumor mill turned with panic of widespread technological disaster and impending world-ending doom and for most IT personnel anywhere, everything changed overnight. Y2K meant working overtime on weekdays and on weekends to make sure this corporation's computers and the end-users were set for the turning of the century. Not only did we have to take care of all this equipment but we had to train key personnel. We worked while the world went crazy.

I started noticing a pattern of increased stress levels, increased incident levels. Along with the predicted technological fall-out came the physical fall-out of my 'stabled-off' condition. It happened when I was on the help desk after 5 p.m. I had been at work since 5:30 a.m. Each person was a 'department'. I was the software testing, installation and configuration department and if my department did not succeed, every other department after me would fail. I loved it. I was always up for the challenge. The department before mine was parts and hardware, after my department was networking. There were only two shifts and we worked around the clock.

Sometimes our responsibilities to meet the Y2K demand caused us to work overlapping schedules in order to meet deadlines. Company executives were extremely demanding and in some cases understandably so. Areas like payroll and benefits were critical. I was saved from the scheduled overlap of the next shift this day because some of the employees failed to ship their computers for software upgrades. I took only two breaks that day. With our workload, the company was lenient and extremely understanding about taking breaks. IT was left alone. We did how we wanted, but we worked because of the demand.

I remember clearing off all the who-knows-what from my workbench. I had all kinds of stuff—from books and laptops to desktops, towers, disks and phones. The room was full of men. I was the ONLY woman in the micro-systems department. The other woman was a manager and was somewhere waiting for one of us to finish or start working on her computer. Executives from other departments were there looking over our shoulders asking questions, trying to get their computers processed first. It was internal company madness. I told the guy next to me that I was out. He looked at me and asked me if I could get *Calgon* to take him away. We both laughed hard. He bid me good night. I stooped down to pick up a stack of five laptops of varying sizes, and when I stood up **blood** ran from the inside of both pant legs and puddled underneath my feet. I was shocked beyond words. I was NOT on my normal IRREGULAR cycle, and there had been absolutely NO incidents at home or in public, and now this. I just stood there, my hands full of laptops. I was supposed to be loading them on the cart to take them to the secure storage area until the following day. The co-worker I'd told I was out for the day was cordial enough that I leaned in his direction.

I didn't dare move either of my feet because the gushing would start so I leaned in as far as I could. I 'bucked' my eyes and most embarrassingly looked down past the laptops still in my hands to where the blood had gone from trickling to slowly running. The blood pool was spreading. He followed my eyes and was smart enough to say, 'Oh God,' in a whisper. I looked at him and urgently whispered for him to give me his jacket and go find another female. He immediately got up and walked over to me without drawing attention to either of us. He acted as though he was helping me when he took the five laptops and gave me his jacket. I tied it around my waist. I looked down at the still spreading pool that was barely hidden by my wide-legged pants. He opened a drawer where we kept paper towels and napkins because sometimes we ate lunch at our workbenches. He just dropped piles of them on the floor in the blood, covering the entire pool but not stooping down to wipe the stuff up. I was just standing there truly embarrassed to the end of the world. He stood in front of me doing all of this.

All the other men were conversing in small groups around the room. All I had to do was make it to the door without someone looking at me. Fortunately, I had on a pair of maroon print pants that didn't allow the blood to show. I stopped being embarrassed long enough to be truly grateful for my co-worker and what he was doing, not to mention how covertly he was doing all of this without me moving. He took one step to stand behind me, holding these laptops, and made it seem as if we were about to secure the laptops or take a break. He said, 'Go,' from behind me and we walked at a normal pace toward the door. There were no turns to get to the door, just a straight shot and I was out. It was what happened when I started walking that almost made me stop. I was trailing blood, long trails of black-red on a stark white polished floor! We kept moving.

After we got outside the door, instead of going to the bathroom down the carpeted hall in this ultra-modern high-rise corporate building, I headed straight for the stairwell down to bathroom on the very next floor. My co-worker's jacket was ruined, and of course I wasn't about to give it back to him. I didn't have a chance to thank him, and I honestly don't know what he did or what happened after I ran out.

I didn't quit this job. I really liked technology and I liked working with men more than women. I never experienced an atmosphere where the guys thought I couldn't hold my own. I was promoted on this job. I stayed there until the next big thing came up for me. My co-worker and I became best friends. He remained a gentleman about everything that happened and we got to take real breaks before I left—but that's another book.

The next-big-thing job was truly that. I was a field tech and a help-desk analyst. This job was mentally demanding and that's an understatement. I was there for several years and every year that I remained at the job I was absent two days every month because of this tormenting issue. I remember coming to work one morning in so much pain my vision would intermittently blur. Putting one foot in front of the other made every bone in my body sting with pain. Somebody told me my eyes were burnt red. I eased around the office call center trying to find the first-aid cabinet and pain medication. I was moving like a snail, whereas I normally walked at breakneck speeds to get anywhere. That was normal for me.

My supervisor, a woman thank God was coming around the corner and I was 'snailing' in her path. As she stepped into the room we came face-to-face. At that moment a jolt worse than any I had previously felt hit my pain-riddled body. I squeezed my eyes shut and physically grabbed my supervisor by the collar of the jacket she was wearing with both hands. My hands fisted tight because I was hurting. I leaned my head on this woman's chest and stayed that way until the pain eased. I inhaled and exhaled once, very slowly. Tears were rolling down my face when I raised my head and hissed, 'Do you have morphine?'

You should have a great supervisor with even greater understanding when things like this happen. My gratitude grew tremendously. I couldn't have been more humble.

My supervisor told me to take the lounge and sent other people and herself moving to find me meds. They returned with the pharmacy at my disposal. My co-workers, supervisors and managers understood that my absence or not moving at my usual lightning pace meant something was wrong. My supervisor signed me out for the next two weeks and emailed an announcement to HR and my field and help-desk teams that I would be out. This was the first of several hospital visits because of this condition. This condition worsened and plagued me throughout my technical career. By now I was a much-sought-after technical professional receiving awards, promotions and raises. The Lord's grace and favor really did go with me everywhere. While I was grateful for everything the Lord had done for me in my career, I decided I wanted to do something different, something to break the tech cycle for a short term. I became a flight attendant and absolutely LOVED flying and all things aviation!

This would have been a productive career change for me had it not been for my constant and vexing companion. This condition was the bane of my blessed existence. By now I was so into flying! Being a newbie meant you got the most grueling schedules, but I loved it. My uniform, hair, nails, everything was crisp, cuffed and creased. My gold wings glowed with my joy, gratitude and pride, and I could serve humanity in the air.

It was short lived. The harder and longer I worked—constantly in the air, the cabin pressure at high altitudes, the long hours and layovers, climbing stairs and running through airports—the worse the situation became. When I thought this condition couldn't get any worse on this beautiful and fun job, I had to call crew scheduling for the same two and three days down time for as long as I was there. This down time became normal and the women in crew scheduling established a code for me. They knew when I called (at certain times each month, though never the *same* time each month). If I had experienced an incident in the air, it would have been bad on so many levels. For those of you that fly, I attended a passenger jet which meant I was the sole flight attendant for more than forty people. When that sole flight attendant has to take a bathroom break on the plane, she has to notify the flight crew. The first officer or an able-bodied passenger has to take over. When this happened I would do airport duty and somebody else would take my flights. That meant having to sit in the airport for up to thirteen hours!

This worked in part because I was always around a bathroom, but I hated being the prisoner of my own body.

I was on the last leg of a six-day flight schedule, coming from Maine to Massachusetts and on to Tennessee. Crew Scheduling called me in Massachusetts and changed my route to Illinois. I had a three-hour layover in Illinois before heading on to Tennessee. It was cold on the northeast coast with snow, high winds and ice. No problem. I always thanked God for safe passage as HE kept us traveling safely through HIS earth and air elements.

As the end of my layover drew closer, I settled into one of the seats at my assigned gate to wait out the thirty minutes. In the cold I wore my military, midnight-blue uniform trench coat. I had my coat on because the airport was chilly. Suddenly I felt hot. I paid no attention to this change but by now I had learned to wear protection on or off dealing with this miserable issue. I knew what it was. I checked in the bathroom just to make sure nothing was untoward. I was good. My plane arrived on schedule, I got my duties taken care of and we were off. It happened in the air—the very worst place.

All that time in the airport and nothing. Now, instead of a trickle or a run, I felt a forceful gushing like having a miscarriage. I was passing huge clots of blood and I couldn't go to the bathroom because we were fifteen minutes from landing and I was about to take my jump seat. I gripped my stomach muscles as hard as I could and sat in that jump seat facing forty-plus passengers. I *invisibly* shook my head. Tightening my abdominal muscles kept a pool from forming on the floor at my feet.

Right before we landed, the captain called back and told me that Crew Scheduling had assigned me one more leg of flying. I was based in Tennessee. Any other time I would have jumped on the extra flight assignment, but this was not that time. A leg is when a plane flies from a scheduled departure station to a scheduled arrival station. Not only did I have an extra leg, but I had to do what is called a 'turn' on this leg, which meant that once I arrived at the scheduled destination, the plane would be prepped to fly out or turn around. When we landed on that portion of the leg in Tennessee, I went to the dugout to call Crew

Scheduling. Getting from the plane through the airport was an incredible feat of continuing to clutch my abdominal muscles while walking at a normal pace ... and dragging three tiers of luggage in my wake. When I got to the dugout, male pilots were everywhere! The ratio of female flight personnel (which includes female pilots) to men is 5 to 100. Blood was starting the path down my pant legs. My uniform was all dark blue and black, except for my startling white shirt—and I didn't have to worry about that.

I had to call from the airport phone because my cell phone battery was dead. I didn't dare plug it into a charging station because that would mean me having to walk through the airport to go upstairs to a certain gate. My protection, which I had checked during my three-hour layover in Illinois, was not protecting me anymore. I didn't have enough money to buy something in the airport. If you fly, you know airport prices are criminally inflated.

A male crew scheduler answered the phone. I asked to speak to a female supervisor. The hour was going on 10 p.m. This meant that most of the familiars who knew my 'code' apparently were not there, and this guy was new. I visibly started shaking my head. I think he purposely gave me a hard time. I asked him several times for a female supervisor. While I was on this call, I was standing with my back toward the open rooms of the dugout where all the pilots were seated. They heard my frustration and vaguely shaded conversation with this hindering person on the phone. Blood was running inside my thick black pantyhose into my shoes. Thank God no one could see this because of my pantyhose. Thank God for my entire uniform and its color. One by one the pilots started walking out as discreetly as they could. After turning around initially and seeing them struggling not to hear me, I didn't turn around again. I helped them help me not to be more embarrassed.

By this time a female supervisor was on a three-way connection with me and the crew scheduler. She knew me. My turn on this leg was canceled and my schedule changed to four days out instead of the regular two. I walked out of the dugout onto the tarmac, to the parking garage and my waiting car. The darkness of my clothes and the night covered me as I drove the interstate stretch home. I was wet underneath and thinking of a hot bath, my bed, clean pajamas and the poor chick that got the call to take my last flight turn in the middle of the night.

———

If you've read through to this portion of the book and are exclaiming how tired YOU are of **reading** about how 'bloody awful' all of this is, then my purpose of enlightening your understanding is being accomplished. Keep in mind, this book is summarizing a twelve-year problem into a few pages and chapters to draw the parallel between two women.

———

By now I'd reached my mid-career stage, and I continued working in corporate America. My next job was a help-desk position where I sat down most of the time. It is a medical fact that sitting for long periods is very stressful to the heart muscle.

Highly stressful jobs were the jobs where I did my best work and received the most awards and promotions. I didn't ask for these kinds of jobs, but they always seemed to be where I ended up. And true to the nature of the 'she-beast', that bloody albatross that continued to hang around my waist in its internal turmoil showed up immediately after lunch one day. Because this was not a physical labor job, I got to wear cute clothes. Not over dressing but ladies, we all understand that sometimes you want to wear a dress or a skirt. My desire to wear a dress or skirt was the same. The skirt I wore was a maxi dark-blue denim pencil skirt.

I only had minimal protection. I could go to the bathroom without incident. As soon and the door to the bathroom closed behind me, I felt my muscles relax and my entire skirt in the back was ruined. I stayed in the bathroom for almost an hour washing and drying my skirt. One of my female co-workers came to check on me. After assessing my situation, we agreed that she would inform our supervisor, who was male, that I was 'ill'. She returned to help me wash and dry my clothes under the hand dryer. This was another time I became grateful for having a few more females working with me. I was saved—sort of—from total public embarrassment that day.

I kept wondering about the circumstances of the woman in the time of Christ. I wondered whether it would have been easier for both of us to have stayed home—her from whatever her daily routine would have been and me from mine. We were both hoping, praying and *reaching* for what we *believed* to be and came to *know* as our ONLY solution.

School Daze

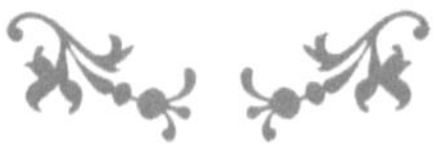

Being in other public places proved no different from being in any of these workplaces; no place or time was off-limits to these embarrassing disasters. Registration day at the university campus left me on the verge of wanting to call the EMTs. I wore a pastel yellow blouse and a stone-washed denim skirt. After a tour of the campus, and before meeting my counselor, I informed my female guide that I was detouring to the ladies' room. She replied where she would be and what would take place on my return. I washed my hands, checked my hair and general appearance in the mirror and was about to walk out the door when blood spread all over the front and the back of my skirt. The spread did not stop there: it also covered one-third of my yellow blouse WITH NO WARNING! No sweating, no pain or cramping, nothing! I stood there watching. It was as though someone was working me over with a paintbrush! It was incredible. The blood appeared in the pattern of an open hand-fan! I thought I was losing my mind.

Someone pushed the door open; it was the guide coming to find out what was taking me so long. I had been in there almost forty-five minutes. She immediately told me she would take care of most of my registration with information she had from our previous phone conversations. I stayed behind to clean up. Nothing pooled at my feet this time but that didn't make it any better. I was beyond embarrassed. The guide and I rushed through the remaining parts of my registration and I went home. Originally, I had signed up to attend classes on campus; after this happened I signed up to take them all online.

The Assurance of Medical Insurance

Coming into the fourth year, I experienced a job loss from corporate America and the loss of my excellent health benefits as well. My husband was working a salary-plus-commission job. The salary was small and the commission was what commission is: a hit-or-miss chance at making extra money. The economic change that took place in my household was a devastating blow.

My physical condition got worse. I could no longer exercise or walk at my optimistic and energetic clip. If I sat down in a chair, getting up would be slow and painful. My bones and joints began to hurt. I felt like I was deteriorating. I could no longer continue visits to my OB-GYN specialist group—and I needed that kind of medical care. My situation was going beyond the threshold of life-threatening.

Even though my physical body was going through these changes, by the grace of GOD my spirit was not subdued. I became more motivated to fight back with THE WORD. Before, I had been caught up with trying to find out WHAT was happening to me and why. Now, I armed myself with the power of the HOLY SPIRIT to ENDURE what I was going through in my body and mind. As it is written, *'The spirit indeed is willing, but the flesh is weak' (Matthew 26:41, KJV).* I started speaking every scripture of healing to my body that I could find. I BELIEVED what I was saying because it was and is THE WORD OF THE LORD. My faith kicked in, and that's when everything became a real battle!

Before I started using THE WORD OF GOD, the physical downward spiral was a situation that started and continued mainly through ignorance and neglect. When I repented of neglecting my body as THE LORD's temple and started fighting back, my body showed signs of responding to GOD'S WORD when I spoke it and believed. When this happened, I decided on doing work-at-home jobs at a time when working from home was being introduced into the workforce as a legitimate option. I had to do something to have medical insurance again, and I turned my mind to TOTAL dependence on GOD. I was blessed with work. I worked for reputable companies. I prayed to the Lord to lead me to reputable online jobs. The Lord NEVER FAILS.

Some of the work-at-home jobs offered medical benefits, but you didn't make enough money from them to take the premiums out of your check. Others didn't offer benefit coverage at all. I realized I should have been more specific with my request and petition to THE LORD about the kind of job that I wanted; nevertheless, I was working. But sitting down all the time proved more detrimental to my uterine condition and my heart.

To Have or Not to Have ... Insurance

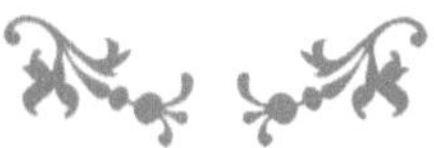

Yes, let's *reeeaaally* talk about health, dental and vision insurance. I mentioned earlier times when I had insurance and times when I did not have insurance. Various medical avenues were or were not available to me depending on what my insurance status was.

One question I believe many people have or may be asking is, 'Why are each of the three components of insurance separate and paid for separately?' And even if others were not asking that question, I asked it continuously. When I was listed under my husband's medical insurance, all three components were listed and labeled MEDICAL INSURANCE. You paid one premium, chose your doctor, dentist or optometrist (in-network, of course), and that was it basically. Also, HMOs made it easy if you had a growing family.

Even now, with the ever-changing insurance markets and the various types of insurance, the question remains, 'Why are all three components not covered under one title, HEALTH INSURANCE?'

According to Nicole Spector, this question is now being addressed ('The Reason Your Dental Work Isn't Covered by Medical Insurance,' *NBC News*, October 25, 2017; retrieved from https://www.nbcnews.com/better/health/reason-yourdentalwork-isnt-coveredmedical-insurance-ncna813666).

When I started having all these problems with AUB, I learned how conditions of the blood and blood flow affect the human body's chemical balance and biological makeup. In my case, my blood levels were consistently low for many years, and this caused me to have tooth decay, hair loss and a gross depletion of vitamins and minerals such as vitamins A, C, D and K, iron and calcium. These vitamins and minerals are major 'building blocks' that give the human body its operational and functional stamina.

The human body depends on the proper blood levels and blood flow. Proper blood flow is vital to maintaining good health and a healthy functioning balance. Also, in **Leviticus 17:11** it is written, *'For the life of the flesh is in the blood ...'* (KJV).

Because there is so much information on health insurance, vitamin and mineral supplements etc., I have listed a few favorite reputable websites:

- https://www.humana.com/all-products/understanding-insurance/hmo-vs-ppo
- https://www.health.harvard.edu/staying-healthy/Listing_of_vitamins
- https://nccih.nih.gov/health/vitamins

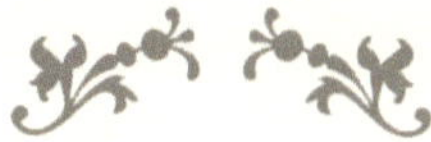

The Question of Disability Benefits

During this time, I filed for disability benefits. I was not well informed about how the process for disability benefits worked or how to apply for them. I just knew I was out of work and my family life and lifestyle were degrading as much as my health. I had to do something to help. You never want to have your family burdened in any way when something causes you to not be able to provide a basic standard of living. Something financially positive needed to happen—and to happen as quickly as possible. I *thought* applying for these benefits would be that something.

I remembered my friend having previously worked in a social security office. She gave me some helpful information about filing for disability. I didn't try to research this on my computer because sitting was a horrible problem and I was in a hurry. Armed with the information I got from my friend, I filed. My husband filled out most of the paperwork sitting next to my bedside. Five or six pages, front and back. I filed using an attorney. I won't go through the entire process in the book but for those of you that have never filed for disability benefits and for those of you that have, I'll just tell you that I was denied. I was shocked. According to the rules of disability eligibility I was qualified but was denied anyway. The filing process, waiting and then being denied took so much more out of me. You have to be dying or dead (obviously a stupidity clause) in order to be approved.

This health issue cycled me through an entire medical community and various medical staff. I believe to this day I was unfairly denied.

The insurance system in this country is absolutely incredible and sometimes incredibly unfair.

Now we have the Affordable Care Act, implemented January 1, 2014. I cannot say if things are better or worse in this country as far as medical insurance is concerned, but I can say—for anyone and everyone that doesn't have medical insurance because of job loss, human disabilities or other reasons—God help us and vote.

Calling Doctor(s) ... STAT!

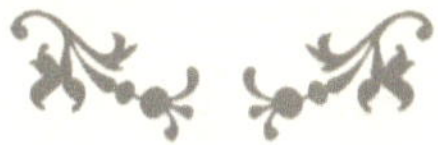

'And had suffered many things of many physicians, and
had spent all that she had, and was nothing bettered,
but rather grew worse ...' Mark 5:26 (KJV)

At the beginning of this book I noted that Luke was one of the three gospel authors inspired to record the **'certain woman's'** condition in the Bible as part of a testament to the healing virtue of Jesus Christ. When I read the verses of scripture about her, I wondered whether Luke was also one of the 'many physicians' that examined her. Was he among the physicians that charged her money? I had so many questions.

One of those questions was, 'Were the physicians of that day prevented from examining this woman because of the Mosaic laws written in *Leviticus* **chapter 15 (KJV)** before Jesus Christ came?'

How did any of the physicians of that day *know* this woman had an issue of blood if the Mosaic laws did not allow them to touch her?

Did this 'certain woman' confide this to the doctors, including Luke, verbally? This was very dynamic to me for so many reasons:

- In the time of Moses, the **Levitical** rule forbade *anyone* from touching a man or woman that had a 'running issue' out of his or her flesh and was rendered 'unclean' *because* of that issue.
- The entire **15th chapter of *Leviticus*** is dedicated to rules and laws

and instructions on how to handle the physical conditions of 'running issues out of the flesh'.

- *Leviticus* 15:19–33 speaks to women that had 'running issues out of their flesh'.

The dynamics that amazed me were how GOD used these laws to contain, treat and handle HIS humanity to eliminate even the symptoms that could cause sickness or disease and the spread of diseases before Jesus Christ came. If a person became ill with a 'running issue' from his or her body, obeying the rules and instructions for how to handle that person would release healing according to the Bible and quarantine the 'running issue'.

The first coming of Jesus Christ eliminated the ritualistic practices of the law. Jesus Christ became the embodiment of the law through HIS grace and HIS healing virtue. Let the church say Amen!

I believe that because of who and what Luke was—a doctor, a scholar and one of the disciples of Jesus—his position and status gave him the best advantage to help this *'certain woman'* find Jesus and be made whole of her plague.

He knew her situation and condition. Both of them, the *'certain woman'* and Luke, knew that Luke (probably) couldn't touch her. I believe she confided her situation to him because he was a doctor and she had to know he was one of the disciples of Jesus.

I believe Luke knew that the only solution he could offer this woman was to tell her about Jesus! He had to know Jesus would be coming to this *'certain woman's'* community. I believe he advised her to make herself available, knowing that there would be a crowd.

Luke may have been the very last of the doctors the *'certain woman'* spoke to before she met Jesus. Remember, she 'spent all her living' on doctors, and of course we all know that when the insurance (in our time) and the money (in any time) runs out, you have to resort to *what and who you know!* This woman knew ***many doctors,*** and I don't believe it was a coincidence that one of those doctors was Luke, a chosen disciple of the ***Savior of the World by whose STRIPES she came to be made HEALED!***

By the time this *'certain woman'* reached Jesus her situation was at its worst.

———

At this point I started researching information on *female* OB-GYN specialists. My earlier checkups had been done by men. I am not male-bashing; I just did not benefit in any way from male doctors, and I did not like them examining me. During the time my condition was worsening and taxing my life, I found MOST of these male doctors did not have the best bedside manner. Some had large, rough hands that were cold when they touched you. In some cases, no care was given to the emotional aspect of the exams at all. Ladies, we know that putting your leg in those cold stainless-steel stirrups makes you shudder and want to push aside the thought of getting a PAP exam.

In my experience with these exams by male OB-GYNs, I felt like insult was added to my injured condition. Their seeming lack of concern for my emotional well-being made me feel as though I was being poked and prodded by robots. Some of these doctors would not give me a detailed diagnosis either. In fact, trying to get a detailed diagnosis was like arm wrestling a bear. The struggle to get information from the examinations was REAL: one-word answers, not facing me or facing me but not looking me in the eye.

There was one male OB-GYN who didn't say a word even when I asked questions! At the end of that exam I felt angry and humiliated, to the point I wanted to kick him in his gonads! He just looked at me, gave me a prescription for pain medication and walked out of the examination room. Well, I knew if I kicked him it would not help my situation and I would probably go to jail and be out of MORE money because of this insensitive excuse for a doctor. Humph.

Another male doctor was a decorated military surgeon. (I made sure this doctor came highly recommended while searching for females in the field.) I was referred to him by an emergency room doctor, also male. This man gave one of the most surprising, almost shocking, responses to examining me that I had ever heard from any doctor, male or female. This highly rated male OB-GYN specialist received information about my horrible condition as a follow-up report from the hospital emergency room. This episode lasted somewhere between twenty-four and forty-eight hours; I came to be in the emergency room because I wouldn't stop bleeding. (I will get into the details of the emergency room experience later in this chapter.)

The follow-up referral was to a well-known OB-GYN clinic that was near me. I remember going into the office and confirming my appointment with the front desk medical staff. I was referred to a female doctor, also highly rated. I was informed about this female doctor by the medical staff as I came into the waiting room outside the exam room. This female doctor asked my name. I answered, and she said, 'Oh, you are the one from the [hospital name] emergency room?' 'Yes, I am.' She then said, 'From Doctor _______?' (she stated the emergency room doctor's name), and again I answered, 'Yes.' She then told me she was not the doctor I was supposed to see and it was time for her to finish her shift for the day. I stood in the doorway looking at her with a poker face. For as many doctors, clinics and hospitals that I had visited, it was unfortunate I got used to experiencing stupidity in the medical field—and sadly this kind of stupidity and negligence ALWAYS comes at a high cost to the patient.

After gathering her belongings and going to the exit door she turned to me and said she would get someone else to examine me.

Enter the military surgeon, asking me the same questions the first follow-up female doctor had. By now I was *sitting* in a chair outside the exam room again. I answered just as I had before. He went to another room to get the faxed report from the hospital. He stood silently reading the entire *two* pages of this report. As he finished, I watched his pupils dilate and his eyes change color. His expression was priceless.

He asked me, 'Are you bleeding now?' I calmly said, 'Yes.' He stared at me, assessing my appearance with an up-and-down motion of his head. I had on a summer sundress of all things, which was bright yellow. (I was fighting depression and wore this bright color instead of black to try and cheer myself up.) I looked the epitome of divine health, from my big beautiful afro to my bright spring-painted toes and sandaled feet: bleeding profusely, continuously in pain and short of breath.

I sat there waiting for this prized military surgeon, who had seen God-knows-what kind of human mutilation on the battlefield, to get over himself. It was ridiculous. Then he said, 'I can't do this. I am not going to examine you.' He started looking around for another doctor, but his feet never moved from where he was standing. 'I am not going to touch *this*,' he said. He continued to refer to the results of the report he had received from the hospital about my condition as *this*. I remained calm. He was upset. The emergency room report stated that my blood levels were at eight the day of my emergency room visit and had risen slightly to ten at this visit. The report that the emergency room doctor sent over to the clinic also stated I needed a blood transfusion *immediately*. All these doctors were passing me over. *I was now sure that my experience mirrored what the **'certain woman'** in Christ's time had experienced. We were **medical outcasts.***

As calm as I was during this visit, I was seething when I got up to leave.

I turned this angry energy into more focused research. I started asking about female OB-GYNs again. I was sick and tired of insensitive, negligent men passing for doctors in the field of obstetrics and gynecology.

It was during this time that I learned so much about why I was NOT having an *irregular period* but **abnormal uterine bleeding.** This dedicated group of OB-GYN specialists was concerned with my total well-being as they explained most compassionately and professionally how I had ended up in such an awful physical place.

They explained how uterine fibroid cysts were a large part of the reason for my pain, constant bleeding and enlarged uterus. Suggestions for and questions about a hysterectomy were given and asked. I researched what a hysterectomy was and why this procedure had been recommended on the website *www.hystersisters.com*. I decided it was not what I wanted at that time. Because the fibroid cysts were in the lining of my uterus, the surgery to remove them would not help my situation. Shortly after, I spoke to a co-worker who had undergone the surgery. After listening to her I was dead set against having a hysterectomy. These doctors honored my wishes and continued to give me the best of care for the next few years.

The third year of my exams with this specialist group brought me back to the consultation table with several doctors. In the consultation I was told I would have to have more than one ultrasound. I was sent to another specialist group for these ultrasound exams and for a second medical opinion. When this was all done the prognosis came in the form of a four-page, certified letter. While I will not share the exact contents of the letter, I will say the contents were not good. The doctors from both specialist groups determined I had three options: an ablation or a partial or total hysterectomy. The letter also told me that because of the AUB, my blood levels were dangerously low and I was in dire need of a transfusion before any surgery could possibly be done. When I sat down for what would be my last consultation with these angels of mercy in human form, I was informed they needed to find a way to keep my blood levels from dropping if I went ahead with any surgery. If my blood levels were kept at a level of between ten and thirteen they could proceed with the surgery.

As I listened to them and understood as they explained everything to me, the entire procedure seemed dangerous and impossible to all of us. At best, it would mean my having to stay in the hospital at least three weeks and not do any physical activity while they made efforts to stop the bleeding and keep my vital signs normal. At worst, it would be a tremendous strain on me and my family and require an incredible arrangement of doctors to get the surgery done. I was stunned! It took me two weeks to show this letter to my husband. After he read it, his reaction was the same as mine during my last consultation with the doctors. I understand why the military doctor told me he would not 'touch *this*': because the danger involved meant finding a way to keep me alive during surgery.

I decided at that time to have the uterine ablation done. According to the American College of Obstetricians and Gynecologists, 'Endometrial ablation destroys a thin layer of the lining of the uterus' *(https:// www. acog.org/Patients/FAQs/Enodometrial-Ablations)*.

I found yet another website that allows you to look up the name, ratings and credentials of your doctors.

I made a first visit to yet *another* OB-GYN group. I chose this specific group for several reasons: it consisted of a diverse group of women, one of these doctors had delivered one of my children and the practice was conveniently located, which meant that I did not have to drive forty-five minutes to an hour across town to get excellent medical care.

As I researched the mission and objectives of this specialist group, one thing stood out for me in what I read: this group was formed and established for the very reasons I stated earlier about male OB-GYN physicians. These were female specialists from around the country. Their credentials were better than good; these were some of the country's best OB-GYN specialists and they were available to me! I was truly grateful for their thoroughness, their compassionate bedside manner and the education I received about women's health. This group cared not only for the physical woman but also about the emotional and mental state of their patients.

I was where I needed to be and I was glad to be there. There was no fear or agitation about being embarrassed or treated with disrespect before, during or after an exam with this group. Nobody had rough or cold hands and the stirrups were cover with warmed crotched socks!

Everything was new and state-of-the-art with this group.

I saw the specialists in this group sporadically for several years. As time continued...so did my condition. As I continued to get checkups during that time, everything changed physically for me under the watchful eye and microscope of these doctors.

The consultations with the doctors of this specialist group confirmed the same diagnosis as the first specialist group. During those consultations, I heard the words 'ablation' and 'hysterectomy' again.

We finalized my decision to go ahead with the ablation.

The word 'destroys' is a very strong word to use to describe a medical procedure relating to this particular problem. I thought so when the word was used in the medical consultations. The lining of the uterus thickens and then sheds during the normal twenty-eight-day menstrual cycle. Well, in the case of AUB, ablation causes the bleeding to pause or causes a prolonged time of not bleeding. For some women with AUB, the ablation actually cures the problem.

After my ablation, the results of the process lasted exactly three months before the AUB returned, just as my job and health insurance ceased ... again.

people they served and the medical staff that served them. These doctors, administrators, accountants, interns and funding agencies were all aligned to the service of economically 'fallen' humanity. For some it was a service much needed, and by me very much appreciated. I honestly can't say that enough. It was like an army of people with the medical knowledge, determination and love for the health and the healing of the sickness and disease of a city whose fight for better health care is a real, continuous struggle.

At this church-supported facility I was given a most disheartening diagnosis: my uterus was now deviated, or curved. As the female doctor told me in consultation, I had now had *TWO* uteruses. Yes, *TWO*. The fibroid tumors that were in the lining of my uterus, as reported to me by the specialist groups, had **grown and separated and would continue to grow.** My body was treating my uterus as if I were pregnant and my blood supply was feeding my uterus as it would a human fetus. I truly had never heard of such a thing! No one could have convinced me I was not in a B-rated horror film!

With every report or diagnosis, things seemed to be spiraling out of reason and my vocabulary was being reduced to the single-word question 'What?'

I was given this information by the doctor as she sat on the front side of her office desk and I sat up close and personally stunned. This is the ABNORMAL part of the uterine bleeding. She gave me an appointment card scheduling me for an endometrial biopsy. She wanted to make sure my reproductive system was not cancerous.

Two weeks later I returned for the biopsy. The doctor told me briefly that a medical intern would be doing the biopsy. Initially I was not comfortable with this but she assured me (when I was hesitant to consent to being examined by an intern) that she would be assisting the entire time with an RN present. I agreed. (This was one of the stupidest decisions I had ever made.)

It was horrible. The procedure probably would have gone very well if the doctor had done my biopsy and not an intern. It took the intern THREE tries before she got the sample!

I sat up in excruciating pain on top of the excruciating pain I was already in. I sat up and for a few moments I let my anger override my pain. I told the intern if she touched me again I would do her bodily harm—and I meant it. I looked at the doctor like I wanted her to feel what I felt but worse. The inside of my body was stinging with pain and blood was squirting from the pressure of me sitting up and the botched biopsy. I felt as though I had become a sacrificial victim in a medieval blood-letting! For the previous two weeks I had been pre-scribed PROGESTIN to slow or stop the bleeding before the biopsy. A lot of good that did! The RN looked as miserable as I felt. I could tell the RN felt like I had been done a medical injustice. Then I looked back at the intern. She looked more miserable than the RN. Her face turned red. I calmed down. This time I let compassion override my anger in response to what I perceived as a sincere silent apology from everyone except the doctor ... who was busy talking to me, maintaining her pro-fessional demeanor and throwing her bedside manner out the window. I mentally added *this* female OB-GYN physician to the 'quack' list of male OB-GYNs. They all left the examining room while I got cleaned up, recovered and dressed. After slowly tipping to her office where all of us gathered for a second time, the doctor told me I needed to have a hysterectomy. She scheduled me for another consultation a week from that time and told me I would be sore for two weeks after this botched biopsy. The inside of my body felt cryptic. When I came back for the consultation the doctor wasn't there. Instead I consulted with the medi-cal director. She told me in no uncertain terms NOT to allow this doctor to schedule me for a hysterectomy. And the reason was that INTERNS would do the entire procedure!

Later I received a letter from the doctor confirming what the medi-cal director told me about interns performing the procedure. I believe to this day that talking to the medical director was divine intervention. One last consultation with the doctor confirmed what I already knew from the medical director: 'Ms. Jamiina, whenever you get health insur-ance again, keep your appointments with me,' she said with a smile. I slowly made my way out of that office and never saw her again.

I went home not knowing what was going to happen now. When I got home I changed my clothes and of course everything else and I sat so quietly in the chair, my husband just looked at me. He knew things had gone badly with the doctor at this urban clinic. He didn't say anything. There was nothing to be said by either of us to the other.

It was then I prayed one of the most **effectual prayers (James 5:16, KJV)** that I had prayed in a long time. I prayed this prayer still sitting in my oversized chair. My head was *not* bowed, my eyes were *not* closed and my mouth *never* opened. *I prayed earnestly from my heart that the LORD please make a way for me to have insurance again. I repented of all arrogance, known or unknown, and of any ungratefulness for previously having health insurance. Not only did I pray for myself but I prayed that the LORD would send more medical personnel, trained and compassionate, into the ripe harvest field of medicine and medical research. I prayed for the intern that did my biopsy. I prayed for anyone wanting to go into any area or field of medicine, whether it be for mental or physical health, that the Lord give them to know and understand this arena was a ministry and they should treat it as an avenue used by GOD to channel HIS healing power.*

I understood that ALL healing comes from GOD and it is our gift from GOD to maintain it. This is how I prayed. Then God gave me HIS peace, to the point I felt sedated. *'The peace of God, which passeth all understanding' (Philippians 4:7, KJV). Then I bowed my head with my eyes closed. I audibly thanked the Lord and fell asleep in my big armchair.*

My Darkest and Daybreak Hour

Several months passed. Nothing. The Lord's peace remained with me. My entire body began to take on a crippled appearance. Nothing stopped the pain. Nothing. I was taking 1,500 milligrams of Naproxen (this made some of my hair fall out) and wearing small hand towels inside the house as extra protection. The only time I went outside was to doctors' appointments, and I carried with me a soft satchel full of towels and plastics just in case.

Now my family had to wait on me hand and foot most of the time. Lots of money was going toward the purchase of laundry detergent, disinfectant, bed clothes and sanitary products. So much money. These purchases became an investment with no financial profit or return. My husband had to buy cases upon cases of feminine hygiene products. I slept in a separate bed from my husband that was covered with plastic and towels. Cloth furniture was replaced with vinyl. I could no longer digest my food because my oxygen supply was short. I would eat very small amounts of soft foods—sometimes baby food—to maintain my body's vitamin intake. I became grossly overweight, most of which was fluid. My body was trying to compensate for the lack of oxygen, which should carry nutrients throughout the body. I would sometimes fall asleep and wake up covered in blue, black and purple bruises and blood. I would groan when I sat down or rose to stand. I had to have help. But this one thing remained: I continued trusting the LORD regardless of what may have happened. I KNEW that HE was still with me.

Many of us have heard the expression 'The darkest hour is just before the dawn'. I believed that phrase was truly descriptive of my situation, and this is where I held on to *Psalm 27:13*: *'I had fainted, unless I had believed to see the goodness of the LORD in the land of the living'* (KJV).

I want to pause and elaborate just a little on EVERYTHING THE LORD opened my eyes to in this ONE scripture, and I'll explain this scripture in segments, the way THE LORD did for me, as I read it for this situation:

1. *(I had fainted)* I NEVER fainted, meaning my body NEVER gave out, because of THE LORD's strength.

2. *(Unless I had believed)* Because I truly learned to TRUST GOD and depend on HIM, HE increased and strengthened my spirit and my faith through HIS WORD.

3. *(To see the goodness of the LORD)* While I did not depend on the doctors, I did see THE LORD's goodness and mercy through them and others. HIS goodness and mercy was truly following me through all of this.

4. *(In the land of the living)* As life-threatening as this situation was—as determined by all the doctors that examined me—I remain(ed) in the land of the living.

Meet the Press with a Stretch of Faith

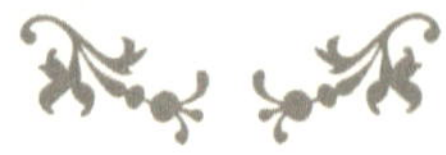

'When she had heard of Jesus, came in the press behind, and touched his garment.' (Mark 5:27, KJV)

Doctors were telling me to eat and drink any and everything that would help generate or strengthen my red blood cells: spinach, beets, small glasses of dark red wine, liver cooked as rare as I could stand it. When I did consume these combinations of iron-producing foods, I felt the results immediately but the positive effects were never lasting. My eyes became extremely sensitive to sunlight. All the shades had to be pulled down in the daytime especially in the summer months. Spurs began to form on the heels of my feet, and walking was brutal—even just taking a few steps. I would walk and rock from side to side just to go from one room to the next and this 'next' room was just the bathroom.

I remember retiring to bed one night and upon waking the next morning my entire body was swollen. I rose swinging my legs over the edge of the bed. My toes touched the floor and pain shot through me like glass bullets. I slid out of bed and crawled quietly wincing, into the bathroom.

I wasn't giving up so I prayed again but I was more specific this time. It was a short prayer asking the Lord to bless me to get complete health insurance after being denied disability insurance. HE answered me. I got the insurance through one of those work-at-home jobs. Yes, I went back to work, sitting. I had to in order to have insurance, since this was the only way I knew to get it. The company was a global company with above-excellent benefits. Insurance coverage was effective on the first day but I was only physically able to work three weeks! I had the means to search for a doctor through the insurance coverage that the LORD provided through this company. The doctor that HE led me to was none other than the doctor that had been a part of the second OB-GYN specialist group—*MY doctor!*

I was shocked and she was so glad to see me. This doctor was no longer a part of that group but was in her own practice. We talked and hugged like we were family. Then we got serious. We covered all the preliminaries. She had my earlier records and recovered the latest ones. I went back and forth from her practice to yet another cardiologist group. They worked another year trying to get my blood levels up. This was truly a vicious medical cycle. Another medical facility was grouped into this 'best of the best'. Newly built and new to my research and knowledge, this hospital had an entire wing dedicated to women's health. The facility covers an area of five city blocks and is built on three levels. The LORD answered my prayers 'exceedingly above all that I could ask or think'.

Over the next few days I was on the phone with my doctor. My daughter walked into the house on one of these days, looked at me and collapsed with joy on hearing that I had been cleared by the cardiologist to have an abdominal hysterectomy. My family had become stressed out after so many years of feeling my pain. Everybody was extremely concerned about all the time that had passed and my encounters with doctors that were afraid to do this surgery. Understanding the potential medical ramifications of the procedure added fear on top of this stress, even for my doctor.

On one of my visits to the new cardiologist my blood pressure went up to 200 over whatever the bottom number was. I started having chest pains so bad that the EKG technician monitoring my heart came in and whispered to the cardiologist, 'She's in a lot of pain.' He didn't know I could hear him. He was right. No one would have known I was in pain because I just lay there, quietly communing with my FATHER (GOD). As soon as I got up the bleeding started. I told the interns that prepped me for the EKG scan and the stress test. I did also inform them that if I were to take this stress test the results would end just as they did, a bloody mess but this time I was prepared.

The technicians called the head cardiologist and I was scheduled to see him the very next day. I was all prepped for this new technical cardio exam. There were two chief cardiologists present while I talked calmly and quietly to the RN who was at my bedside. I saw the cardiologists were reading my information on the charts and files. One cardiologist said, 'Ms. Jamiina, myself and Dr. So-and So saw you for this same problem ten years ago.' I turned my face to the wall and cried. The RN almost cried too.

The nurses came and ministered to me. Then the cardiologists said, 'We're going to take care of *this … this* time, don't worry.' They ran more tests. I got dressed and was told that I should come back in two weeks and that I would get the results of these tests in three or four days.

This testing back and forth between the OB-GYN and the cardiologist continued. It was incredibly costly and time-consuming. It took so much out of my life and my time with my family.

The severity of my low blood levels was the reason that I had to have cardiologists, but I didn't realize I had to have a **team** of them. My low blood levels caused my heart to beat harder and later caused my heart to develop the previously mentioned murmur.

The cardiology team had to send a letter to clear me to have surgery. They were all aware of the possibility of my 'expiring' during any surgical procedure.

In October of that year, the OB-GYN was able to get my blood level up to thirteen. The normal level should be thirty.

We were all hopeful about this. We waited three weeks and the surgery for the hysterectomy was scheduled. Or so we thought. During the last three days of those three weeks my blood levels plummeted. I soon found myself being swept through a doorway by three very tall and very strong nurses. The scene looked like something from a popular television show about an army mobile hospital unit. I remember before they swept in I had been talking to one of the RNs. As I sat in front of her desk answering questions I was keenly aware of all the hubbub around me. I saw nurses in a colorful swirl of hospital scrubs fluttering and scurrying in every direction, but mostly concentrated around me. I turned my focus back to the head nurse at the desk in front of me. The next two statements that came out of her mouth made me think that this was a good time for me to show some optimism and enthusiasm. (I didn't feel optimistic or enthusiastic.) This nurse looked up at me and seemed to be extremely serious about *something*. She asked me, 'Ms. Jamiina, did you know your blood levels were extremely low?' I said, 'Yes.' She then asked, 'What happened to your blood, where did it go?' To me this was a stupid question because I thought the medical staff was supposed to know this and tell *me* what had happened to my blood. I thought she was joking so I decided to try my brand of slapstick comedy.

Doing my best to be funny in this stressful situation I answered, 'Vampires?' This nurse looked at me and her face turned so red she looked sunburned. She frowned at me and flipped the clipboard with the record of my vital signs and blood levels to one of the other nurse 'flurries' fluttering and hovering behind her. That is when the nurses rushed me from behind lifted me from the chair with my feet clear of the floor and rushed me to an emergency prep room. The nurse 'flurries' had turned into a team of medical stormtroopers. I thought I would have been given a prescription, told to get dressed, go home and start the exams over the next day. I had become used to that process. Instead I was moved from the emergency prep room, where I was asked questions like 'How many fingers do you see?' and 'Who is the president of the United States?', to the women's clinic section of the hospital. For what seemed like an hour I just watched the hospital staff do their daily operations and wondered why I was still there. I didn't remember being in any pain. Suddenly the fluttering started again. I watched and waited. When the cloud of nurses cleared my view and I could see beyond the foot of the bed, my OB-GYN doctor came to my bedside. This was the first time I had seen her since the exams began with the cardiologists. I was so grateful to have her there. I asked, 'What's up with all the commotion?' This compassionate, funny and absolutely wonderful doctor leaned over the bed railings and said, 'Well, with your blood levels and you constantly bleeding we don't want to release you, and we can't do this procedure here because we are not equipped for surgery on this side of the hospital. We have to move you to the other side.'

For some reason all this information she gave me continued not to register so I asked another question. 'Okay, so how serious is it, Doc?' I was ready to get back to the house so I could get in my own bed and get some sleep. My doctor leaned further over the hospital bed railings, inches from my face and said, 'Your situation is acute and we have to move you to the section of the hospital where there are supplies of blood on hand as we go into surgery.' Then she steepled her fingers, leaned closer and said, 'Jamiina, if something were to happen during surgery your body does not have a blood reserve to compensate and you would expire immediately.'

My comedy dead-panned.

Before I could form a decent sentence, the hospital intercom system crackled, *'Calling Dr. One, Dr. Two, Dr. Three and Dr. Four (my doctor) ... STAT!'* My doctor left my bedside, but not before giving me a very reassuring touch on the hand.

For a few moments after she left, the room was empty. No nurses, no commotion, just quiet. I became more sleepy. Just as I was about fall asleep sitting up, I saw this male doctor (I knew he was a doctor because he had on solid blue scrubs) pacing at the foot of the bed I was in. Back and forth. He looked really strange to me—either he was strange looking or I was more tired than I thought. He was short, about 5'7", wearing royal blue scrubs. His hair was really thick and stuck out from beneath the surgical cap. His hair was dark brown, like a child's crayon color and he had on black 1950s plastic-framed glasses with thick lenses. Then I noticed not only was he in scrubs but he had on the surgical mouth guard which hung down around his neck. He looked as though he had just come from surgery or was getting ready for surgery and all he had to do was scrub up.

He paced and looked at me, never saying a word. I shook my head. I was thinking, 'I hope this quack is not taking *my doctor's* place. Here I am in the company of another one of those medical idiots that does not have the decency to speak.' I wanted to throw my shoes at him. I won't apologize for thinking badly of him because anybody with speech can speak and it was obvious he chose not to. His pacing had a buzzard-like quality. An RN came in and informed me I was about to be moved. She asked if I felt like walking to the other side of the hospital or did I need a wheelchair. I actually wanted to walk clean out of the hospital and back home. As I accepted the wheelchair the buzzard continued his back-and-forth pacing at the foot of the bed. As we were leaving and almost through the double doors to the other side of the hospital this idiot yelled out, 'Ms. Jamiina, I hope you make it!' If spit were a brick I would have aimed right between his eyes!

> *'Daughter, thy faith hath made thee whole; go in peace,*
> *and be whole of thy plague.'* (Mark 5:34, KJV)

After my doctor got clearance to do the surgery from the cardiologist, my poor family worried more. My daughter was so afraid for me. My husband started chain smoking but he would never say anything. When they got the surgery date, my daughter kept asking more than ever whether I was scared or nervous. My husband just kept looking at me and not saying anything. All this kept up for the three weeks until the surgery day. Twenty-four hours before surgery I went back to my 'prayer closet'. I had been praying from my hospital bed but this day I crumpled down on my knees and then stretched out prostrate to pray. I didn't bow down for myself; I bowed down for my poor family. Jesus, please! I was truly at peace about my surgery. When I was raised by my family's helping hands off my face, I opened my Bible. THE LORD spoke to me through HIS word and the scriptures spoke of my outcome during and after surgery. I told and showed my daughter what the scriptures said. My body stopped hurting that same day—and this was a day before surgery. My husband listened from the across room, still not saying anything, but he stopped chain smoking. My daughter was apprehensive until the doctor called. I put the doctor on speaker.

My family heard the doctor say, 'Jamiina, I have been praying because of the nature and seriousness of this procedure and because it made me nervous for you but I have peace now and we are going to do this!' And, yes, I truly had a praying doctor!

Her statement was a confirmation and a declaration in the same breath. God is awesome!

My daughter and husband both exhaled sighs of genuine relief. It was as though a stone had been lifted from all our lives.

As it was with the *'certain woman'* some two thousand years ago, as recorded in the scriptures and **verse 28 *of Mark* chapter** 5*: "If I may but touch the hem of HIS garment, I shall be made whole." (KJV)* so it came to be with me.

Through prayer and *FAITH* in the WORD and power of GOD, we received my ***complete*** healing started with trusting HIM and the first manifestation of that healing was the PEACE of GOD we all received and embraced.

The next day it seemed like EVERYBODY that waited on us *knew* us. I know that hospital staff are alerted and are supposed to know who is arriving for any procedure, but this was like being welcomed instead of being acknowledged. The compassion almost brought tears to my eyes. It started with the hospital representative that got my insurance information.

After I was prepped for surgery, we waited. My husband asked me whether I was okay, and I just looked at him like, 'Really?'—but it was a look that said to him, 'You know it's okay.' He smiled.

My doctor's medical team was there, talking, joking and introducing themselves and briefing me on their roles in the procedure. The cardiologists were in the hospital on standby.

Then my doctor showed up. From across the room everyone turned as the door opened. She stood there for a few moments and looked at me. Everybody was quiet. She asked how I felt as she acknowledged her team (the respect everybody showed her was royal and she was so down-to-earth) and explained that she was a bit late because she wanted to make sure the letter of clearance for surgery was there from the cardiologists.

Sitting on the bed that I lay in, my doctor said, 'Jamiina, I was really worried about you and about doing this procedure but seeing you this morning and how you are ... We are going to be alright.'

My doctor wanted to know if I was nervous. All of us had been through a lot. When she asked how I was again, I held out both my hands to show my steadiness and inner calm. I told her that I had prayed the night before and that the words she had said to me on the phone were a confirmation of how things would go. I even told her the scriptures because I had not mentioned this before, I was making sure of my family.

She turned to her team and said, 'Let's go,' quietly but with the command of a military general.

At that moment the room turned a blinding white and instead of a medical team in their colorful scrubs, every last one of them seemed to be dressed in all white robes and my doctor appeared to be wearing a sterling silver suit of armor with a sword in her hand. It was amazing!

Please keep in mind, no meds or anesthesia had been administered at this point. But I understood that the LORD had changed my view to see them that way to assure me HE was there. Just like HE said HE would be in HIS confirmed word. Blessed be the NAME OF THE LORD.

The next time I heard or saw anything I was in a recovery room and my husband was sitting at the foot of my bed watching TV. I felt extremely sleepy and there was something warm and very comfortable on my legs underneath the covers. I drifted off again and then I heard my doctor come in. I asked were we ready for surgery. She laughed a hearty laugh, grabbed both my hands and said, 'Dear, the surgery is over. How do you feel?'

I was shocked. I looked at the foot of the bed and at my husband as he answered, 'You didn't know anything.' He and my doctor laughed at me and it was great to hear. My doctor told me about the procedure. She said she had made a six to eight inch horizontal incision at the base of my abdomen to remove my uterus. Then she made a weird statement describing the physical appearance of the removed uterus. She said, 'It was pretty ugly; it look liked the head of Medusa.'

Of course, this statement cleared my head of any remaining medicinal fog. I frowned when I looked at her. She laughed and said, 'I say "pretty ugly" because the beauty is that your uterus was not cancerous. The ugliness was the numerous fibroids and the size of it was like nothing that I've seen in all my years of gynecology.'

My doctor checked the incision and continued talking with this wonderful bedside manner and genuine smile. 'This incision looks great,' she said, as if she didn't know her own work. She gave glory to GOD as she walked out of the room, relieved and leaving behind a sleepy and grateful patient.

All Things New

When I came into my doctor's new practice for my follow-up exam there were new faces that I didn't recognize from the time of my first visits. I informed the receptionist of my appointment. After the receptionist heard my name she asked, 'You're Jamiina Lynn?' I said, 'Yes,' and began wondering if there was a problem. Her facial expression was classic and as I watched her eyes tear up, she stepped away from the desk and gave me a most compassionate hug. Then she turned still holding my arm and called some of the other staff to meet me. They finally told me my doctor had spoken to them about my entire ordeal. The remaining staff members started hugging me; some were crying, others were crying and smiling. (All were women.)

I cried too, as everyone expressed to me their understanding of my ordeal and the seriousness of what I had been through. I wasn't ready for such a reaction. I certainly didn't know I was going to be met with this reception but it made me feel most human. I don't know if I could have been more grateful at any other time before this. My doctor finally came out and the small crowd parted to make room for her in the circle.

With her down-home perfect Southern hospitality she laughed and told everybody again, 'I was really scared for myself and for you Jamiina. I had to talk this through with my staff and have them pray for me and you the entire time.' When she made this statement this time I realized that my doctor had been depending SOLELY on THE LORD for success with the surgery!

Then everybody laughed with so much relief as GOD continued to get the glory for what HE alone had done through the people of HIS choosing.

Epilogue

*Some would argue the power of GOD and not accept or believe that HE would use or work his healing virtue through medicine or even through people but to that I say, "**The earth is the LORD's and the fullness thereof; the world and they that dwell therein**" (Psalms 24:1, KJV). This experience has taught me how to trust the LORD and truly submit to HIM and not concern myself with the process that HE uses to bring about the blessings that HE so graciously bestows on us. "**And there are differences of administrations but the same Lord**" (1 Corinthians 12:5, KJV).*

When we learn to trust HIM, we witness HIS WORD fulfilled in our lives and we experience abundance in life and provision.

From a 'certain woman' and her physician, a disciple of THE MESSIAH, two thousand years ago, to a certain woman and her Christian physician in the twentieth and twenty-first centuries ...

*Two women, two doctors, same plague ... "**One Lord, one faith, one baptism**" (Ephesians 4:5, KJV).*

*"**Jesus Christ the same yesterday and to day and for ever**" (Hebrews 13:8, KJV).*

For anyone and everyone reading this book, I pray that by it you are encouraged to seek THE LORD for salvation, deliverance and healing from any illness or adversity in your life and come to KNOW HIM as your personal SAVIOR. Amen.

www.ingramcontent.com/pod-product-compliance
Lightning Source LLC
Chambersburg PA
CBHW051416250726
48655CB00003B/1083